Colloidal Silver

A Beginner's Quick Start Guide and Overview on its Use Cases, with an FAQ

mf

copyright © 2022 Felicity Paulman

All rights reserved No part of this book may be reproduced, or stored in a retrieval system, or transmitted in any form or by any means, electronic, mechanical, photocopying, recording, or otherwise, without express written permission of the publisher.

Disclaimer

By reading this disclaimer, you are accepting the terms of the disclaimer in full. If you disagree with this disclaimer, please do not read the guide.

All of the content within this guide is provided for informational and educational purposes only, and should not be accepted as independent medical or other professional advice. The author is not a doctor, physician, nurse, mental health provider, or registered nutritionist/dietician. Therefore, using and reading this guide does not establish any form of a physician-patient relationship.

Always consult with a physician or another qualified health provider with any issues or questions you might have regarding any sort of medical condition. Do not ever disregard any qualified professional medical advice or delay seeking that advice because of anything you have read in this guide. The information in this guide is not intended to be any sort of medical advice and should not be used in lieu of any medical advice by a licensed and qualified medical professional.

The information in this guide has been compiled from a variety of known sources. However, the author cannot attest to or guarantee the accuracy of each source and thus should not be held liable for any errors or omissions.

You acknowledge that the publisher of this guide will not be held liable for any loss or damage of any kind incurred as a result of this guide or the reliance on any information provided within this guide. You acknowledge and agree that you assume all risk and responsibility for any action you undertake in response to the information in this guide.

Using this guide does not guarantee any particular result (e.g., weight loss or a cure). By reading this guide, you acknowledge that there are no guarantees to any specific outcome or results you can expect.

All product names, diet plans, or names used in this guide are for identification purposes only and are the property of their respective owners. The use of these names does not imply endorsement. All other trademarks cited herein are the property of their respective owners.

Where applicable, this guide is not intended to be a substitute for the original work of this diet plan and is, at most, a supplement to the original work for this diet plan and never a direct substitute. This guide is a personal expression of the facts of that diet plan.

Where applicable, persons shown in the cover images are stock photography models and the publisher has obtained the rights to use the images through license agreements with third-party stock image companies.

Table of Contents

Introduction	6
What Is Colloidal Silver?	8
History of Colloidal Silver	10
The First Few Years	10
A Revival in the Most Recent Years	11
Silver in Chemistry	12
Background of Silver	13
Different Forms of Colloidal Silver	15
How does colloidal silver work?	19
Potential Benefits of Colloidal Silver	21
Potential Use Cases of Colloidal Silver	23
Potential Risks and Side Effects of Colloidal Silver	33
Who should not use colloidal silver?	38
Government's Reactions to Colloidal Silver	42
Conclusion	45
FAQ About Colloidal Silver	48
References and Helpful Links	50

Introduction

You may have noticed goods containing colloidal silver on sale either online or in physical places. They are available in a variety of forms, including liquids, gels, and sprays, among others.

Some individuals are under the impression that taking colloidal silver can assist in strengthening the immune system, warding off infections, enhancing circulation, and reducing inflammation. Even if there is no proof from scientific research to back these claims, there are still some people who swear by their efficiency.

It is stated that colloidal silver is an effective antibacterial agent, and it may be applied locally to heal wounds or taken orally to cure stomach ulcers. Both of these treatments are viable options. Even though there is no empirical proof to back these claims, many individuals continue to use colloidal silver as a home cure despite this fact.

However, it is essential to be aware of the potential negative consequences that may arise from the use of colloidal silver. If it is not utilized appropriately, colloidal silver might pose health risks. When used orally, it has the potential to induce nausea, vomiting, diarrhea, and damage to the kidneys. Additionally, it can have an antagonistic influence on the way some drugs work by interacting with them.

Additionally, colloidal silver has been shown to induce a skin discoloration known as argyria. This condition is permanent and cannot be reversed, so it can have a significant impact on how you look. If you are thinking about utilizing colloidal silver, it is essential that you first discuss this possibility with your healthcare professional.

In this introduction to colloidal silver, we'll concentrate on the following subtopics for a more in-depth discussion:

- What is Colloidal Silver?
- History of Colloidal Silver
- Background of Silver
- Different Forms of Colloidal Silver
- How does colloidal silver work?
- Potential Benefits of Colloidal Silver
- Potential Use Cases of Colloidal Silver
- Potential Risks and Side Effects of Colloidal Silver
- Who should not use colloidal silver?
- Government's Reactions to Colloidal Silver

Keep reading to learn more about colloidal silver.

What Is Colloidal Silver?

A colloid is a combination of two substances, often liquids, in which one component of the blend is broken up into extremely minute bits and distributed throughout the other components of the mixture. The bigger particles are known as the suspending medium, while the smaller particles are referred to as colloids. The substance known as colloidal silver is an example of a colloid. It consists of very small particles of silver that are suspended in water. Because the pieces of silver are so tiny, they can float freely in the liquid, creating a suspension that gives the impression of being silver in color.

Silver is a metal that is normally found in its purest form, which is a white metal that has a tint of blue in it. In addition to having the highest electrical conductivity, it also boasts the highest reflectivity of any metal. Silver is a versatile material that may be used for a wide variety of purposes due to its antibacterial qualities as well as its other beneficial features.

Coins, jewelry, and a variety of other items have been crafted with their use going back centuries. Mirrors, photography, and electrical connections and conductors are some of the other modern applications for silver. Even its potential application in the filtration of water and as an antibacterial agent is currently the subject of research.

Colloidal silver has a long history of usage as a traditional treatment for a variety of illnesses and ailments. Several people assert that it may strengthen your immune system, help you fight infections, and even treat cancer. Colloidal silver may be produced in a variety of quantities and forms, including sprays and droplets, for example.

Oral consumption, either in the form of a beverage or a supplement pill, is possible. Additionally, it may be administered to the skin in its purest form. However, there is no scientific evidence to support either the safety or usefulness of using colloidal silver to treat any ailment.

History of Colloidal Silver

The First Few Years

Ancient Greeks were the first people to employ colloidal silver for therapeutic purposes. Silver solutions were used to cure wounds and ulcers by Hippocrates, who is considered the father of medicine. Colloidal silver was widely used beginning in the early 1900s, which is considered to be more recent in history. As was stated before, it was manufactured by pharmaceutical firms and distributed under a variety of brand names, such as Protargol and Argyrol.

These remedies were utilized in the treatment of several ailments, including but not limited to acne, pink eye, and sinus infections. Unfortunately, because of the exorbitant cost of manufacture, it could only be used on patients with a significant amount of wealth. In the 1930s, the discovery of quick-acting and less expensive medications such as sulfa medicines and penicillin led to a reduction in the use of colloidal silver as a medical treatment.

A Revival in the Most Recent Years

Colloidal silver has been making a comeback in recent years after experiencing a decrease in popularity in the middle of the 1900s. This is probably because it is effective against a diverse assortment of bacteria, viruses, and fungi. In addition to this, colloidal silver is safe to consume and does not result in any unpleasant side effects, unlike certain conventional antibiotics.

Even for use as a disinfectant in hospitals and other medical facilities, the EPA has given colloidal silver its stamp of approval. This is because it can eliminate germs and viruses that are present on surfaces without causing any harm to either people or animals. It should come as no surprise that colloidal silver is gaining popularity as an alternative to conventional antibiotics, given the lengthy history of its application and the efficiency with which it has been demonstrated.

Silver in Chemistry

The chemical symbol for silver is Ag, and its atomic number is 47. Silver is a precious metal. Silver is a transition metal that is soft, white, and shiny. It is found in the crust of the Earth in very modest quantities, and it is almost always found coupled with other elements such as sulfur, arsenic, antimony, or chlorine.

Silver is a valuable metal that may be utilized in several different contexts. In terms of optical reflectivity, it is second only to mercury, and it has the lowest contact resistance of any metal. It has the highest electrical and thermal conductivity of any element, and it is the most reflective element. Silver is utilized in water purification systems as well as medical devices due to its inherent ability to inhibit the growth of microorganisms.

In addition, silver nanoparticles may be found in a wide range of products, such as paints, coatings, and textiles. In addition, silver ions are employed in food packaging to suppress the growth of germs and increase the shelf life of the product. In addition, silver acts as a catalyst in a wide variety of chemical processes, including the Haber-Bosch process, which is used to produce ammonia.

Ever since ancient times, people have placed a high value on silver, and its uses continue to develop even in this day and age. It is a flexible component that may be utilized in a wide variety of settings, ranging from the medical industry to the electrical industry and beyond. Due to the one-of-a-kind qualities it possesses, silver has tremendous untapped potential.

Background of Silver

For almost two thousand years, silver has been utilized in the medical field. Ancient peoples from all over the world, including the Greeks, Egyptians, and Romans, utilized silver as a means to improve immune system performance and forestall the deterioration of food and water. Hippocrates, the "father of medicine," is credited with having written in his medical books that silver has great healing and disease-preventing powers.

During the Middle Ages, affluent godparents would gift silver spoons to their godchildren as a baptism present. The spoons would be used to feed the child. In the era before the development of antibiotic medications, silver was one of the few antibacterial remedies that could be utilized. It was utilized in the treatment of skin ulcers, wounds, sutures, syphilis, and infections that occurred after birth in newborns.

In 2015, NASA gave its blessing to the installation of a water filtration system that utilizes silver onboard the International Space Station. This method eliminates the requirement for the use of chemicals or filtration systems by killing bacteria and other germs in water with the help of silver nanoparticles.

There is some evidence to suggest that silver may be beneficial in killing drug-resistant bacteria such as MRSA, however, more research needs to be done in this area (methicillin-resistant Staphylococcus aureus). In addition to that, research is being done on its potential applications in wound dressings and as an antibacterial coating on various medical equipment.

Different Forms of Colloidal Silver

Colloidal silver is offered for purchase in a wide variety of formats, such as ointments, drops, and sprays, amongst others. It is also attainable in the form of liquid or capsules to be consumed orally. While some colloidal silver products are created by the use of electricity (electrolysis), others are manufactured through the use of chemical processes.

Drops

Colloidal silver drops are the most popular kind of colloidal silver, and you can find them simply at health food stores or on the internet. They are easy to employ, and one has complete command over the dose they deliver. Colloidal silver drops include extremely minute particles of silver, which makes it simple for the body to take them in and use them.

Additionally, colloidal silver drops have a lengthy shelf life and may be kept at room temperature without losing any of their properties. On the other hand, many think the taste of the colloidal silver drops is unpleasant. Additionally, because the particles in colloidal silver drops are so minute, they can quickly enter the bloodstream and build up in the body over time, which can result in negative side effects such as argyria.

Sprays

Sprays are generally used for wounds as well as skin infections when using a spray. They also have applications in the nares and the eyes. The use of a spray has the benefit over the use of other forms, such as creams or gels, in that it can reach areas that other forms cannot. Because of this, it is an efficient method of therapy for places that are difficult to access.

Ointments

Due to the antibacterial characteristics of colloidal silver ointments, they are efficient in treating wounds and promoting the body's natural ability to repair itself. The ointments have a basis of petroleum jelly, beeswax, or shea butter, which helps to protect the skin while the silver does its work. This is done so that the skin can better absorb the benefits of the silver.

Ointments containing colloidal silver can be used directly on wounds such as cuts, scrapes, and burns to aid in the prevention of infection and the promotion of healing. Colloidal silver in the form of an ointment is popular among those who are seeking an efficient approach to treating small injuries since it is simple to apply and offers a high degree of convenience.

Capsules

Taking colloidal silver in the form of capsules is a convenient alternative to the traditional method of mixing it with other liquids to get the advantages of colloidal silver. You may get them at health food stores as well as on the internet.

Silver water

The production of silver water involves the addition of silver nanoparticles to water that has been distilled or filtered. The nanoparticles of silver are dispersed throughout the water but do not sink to the bottom. Antiseptic properties are attributed to silver water, which contains a significant number of nanoparticles of silver in high concentrations.

To cure wounds, burns, and infections, silver water is typically employed. Additionally, it is utilized in the cleansing of water. To disinfect medical equipment, institutions like hospitals and clinics may sometimes use silver water. Additionally, it is utilized in the industrial sector to cleanse water before it is put to use in electronic apparatus.

Bandages and dressings

Bandages and dressings containing silver are non-toxic, making them suitable for use on both adults and children; also, they are simple to apply to the skin. Bandages and dressings that include silver are available in a wide variety of sizes and forms, which enables their application to any portion of the body. They have the potential to aid in the prevention of infection and the acceleration of wound healing.

Nebulizer

It is believed that nebulized colloidal silver is effective in reducing inflammation and destroying bacteria and other pathogens that may be present in the lungs. In addition to that, there are assertions that it strengthens the immune system. Nevertheless, there is not a single piece of scientific data to back up these statements.

Lotion

On the market, you may find a wide variety of silver-based lotions, each with its specific purpose. These may be used to treat a variety of skin diseases, including eczema, psoriasis, acne, and rashes since they have been made with several different substances. It is believed that colloidal silver when applied directly to the skin, has a minor therapeutic effect that can assist in lowering inflammation and increasing the body's natural ability to repair itself.

Products containing colloidal silver are promoted for sale as homeopathic remedies. Homeopathy is not considered to be an independent medical system, nor is it acknowledged by the scientific community as a viable therapeutic option.

Before taking colloidal silver or any other homeopathic cure, it is essential to discuss the treatment with your primary care physician, just as it is with any other homeopathic medication. You should also be aware that ingesting an excessive amount of colloidal silver might result in major health complications.

How does colloidal silver work?

Silver is known to be effective against a wide variety of microorganisms, including fungi, viruses, and bacteria.

When colloidal silver is consumed, the silver particles pass past the stomach and attach to proteins in the blood. This prevents the silver from being absorbed into the body. The silver particles are carried through the circulatory system and distributed to a variety of organs and tissues, where they come into touch with microorganisms such as bacteria, viruses, and fungi.

These bacteria serve as the target for the ions of silver, which stop them from multiplying and spreading further. In addition, the bacteria' metabolisms are disrupted by the silver ions, which results in the microbes losing their ability to produce energy and eventually dying.

Colloidal silver contains ions of silver, which, when applied topically, can aid in the battle against skin infections. In addition to this, they can decrease inflammation and hasten the healing of wounds.

In a nutshell, colloidal silver has been utilized for the treatment of bacterial, viral, and fungal illnesses for a considerable amount of time. Because it possesses antibacterial characteristics, silver is efficient against a wide variety of different kinds of microbes. Colloidal silver is making a resurgence in recent years because it is beneficial and does not have any negative side effects. Although further research is required to discover colloidal silver's full potential, there is reason to be optimistic about its potential as an alternative to conventional antibiotics.

Potential Benefits of Colloidal Silver

Many people use colloidal silver as a home cure since it is said to have a variety of positive effects on one's health. It is held by some to be able to strengthen the immune system, aid in the battle against infections, and even assist in the reversal of some chronic disorders. Just a handful of the many advantages of colloidal silver are listed here.

Increases the Function of the Immune System

One of the primary advantages of colloidal silver is that it can assist in increasing the functionality of the immune system. Colloidal silver is an effective antibacterial agent that can eradicate pathogenic bacteria, viruses, and fungi. Because of this, it is a good therapy for ailments such as the common cold, influenza, and even certain forms of infections. It is possible to strengthen your immune system using colloidal silver by eliminating germs and assisting your body in its battle against infection.

Reduces Inflammation

Colloidal silver, a popular alternative treatment that is thought to offer several health advantages, is one of the ways that inflammation may be reduced. One of the most important claims made about it is that it can assist in the reduction of inflammation. When the body is hurt or attacked by an illness, its natural defense mechanism is inflammation.

Reduces Pain

Colloidal silver is believed to be an effective remedy for pain alleviation. It has long been used to treat various kinds of aches and pains, from joint pains to headaches. Several studies have shown that it is capable of reducing inflammation, which could help reduce the intensity of the pain.

On the other hand, persistent inflammation can result in several other health concerns. Because of its anti-inflammatory qualities, colloidal silver may be able to assist in bringing about a general reduction in inflammation throughout the body.

Promotes Healing

Colloidal silver's capacity to promote healing is the most persuasive proof for its purported health benefits, even though some anecdotal data exists to back up these claims. Colloidal silver is a useful therapy for wounds, burns, and skin disorders such as eczema and psoriasis because it can help decrease inflammation and encourage the creation of new cells.

There is some evidence to suggest that colloidal silver can be an effective natural cure for a range of diseases and disorders; however, further study is required to verify these claims. It has a long history of usage as a traditional treatment, and in recent years, its popularity has been growing because it is beneficial while also having no negative side effects. If you are seeking a natural treatment for several ailments, you might want to give some thought to colloidal silver as an alternative therapy option.

Potential Use Cases of Colloidal Silver

It is claimed that colloidal silver, which is a suspension of silver particles in a liquid, is efficient against more than 650 different types of bacteria, viruses, and fungi. Many diseases, including the common cold, influenza, pink eye, and sinus infections, can be treated with colloidal silver, and its proponents utilize it for this purpose. It is also supposed to aid in the healing of wounds, as well as treat ear infections, acne, and yeast infections.

Cold and influenza

Colloidal silver is a common home medicine used to cure a variety of respiratory illnesses, including the common cold and influenza. Colloidal silver, which consists of silver particles dispersed in water, is thought to be effective because it binds to the proteins found in viruses, leaving the viruses harmless. Some individuals think that colloidal silver can be useful in treating and preventing the common cold and influenza, even though there is no scientific evidence to support these claims.

Infections of the skin

Colloidal silver is a common treatment used at home to treat infections of the skin. It is said to be effective in treating a variety of skin disorders, including but not limited to wounds, ulcers, eczema, psoriasis, acne, and ringworm. There are a variety of topical applications for colloidal silver, including soaps, gels, sprays, and creams. There is some evidence to support the use of colloidal silver for the treatment of skin infections; however, there is very little scientific data to back up these claims.

Insect bites

Some individuals believe that bug bites may be treated with colloidal silver, whereas others do not. As a result of its anti-inflammatory effects, it is supposed to minimize the pain, swelling, and itching that are associated with being bitten by a bug. Some people think that colloidal silver can give relief from the discomfort that is associated with bug bites. However, there is no scientific evidence to support these claims.

Ear infections

Because colloidal silver is known to help decrease inflammation and kill germs, it has the potential to be used as a therapy for ear infections. Nevertheless, to verify these effects, further study is required.

Yeast infection

Colloidal silver is a common treatment used in homes across the country for the treatment of yeast infections. When applied to the skin, it has the potential to provide relief from both itching and burning. In addition, there is some evidence that using colloidal silver can assist in reducing the amount of vaginal discharge.

According to the findings of several studies, colloidal silver may be able to assist in the destruction of yeast cells. Despite this, further research is required to substantiate these findings. If you have a yeast infection and are considering utilizing colloidal silver as a treatment, you should first consult with your primary care physician. They can assist you in weighing the dangers of the therapy against its potential advantages and determining whether or not it is the treatment that you should pursue.

Sinus infections

Infections of the sinuses are a frequent condition that afflicts millions of individuals each year. Sinus infections can be treated with antibiotics. Even while antibiotics are typically effective in treating them, there are still many who would rather look for alternative solutions.

One of these remedies, known as colloidal silver, is reported to be useful in the treatment of sinus infections. This is because it possesses antibacterial qualities, which aid in the destruction of the bacteria that are the root cause of sinus infections. Additionally, colloidal silver can assist in the reduction of inflammation and hasten the body's natural ability to repair itself.

Pink eye

For hundreds of years, colloidal silver has been used as a treatment for pink eye, also known as conjunctivitis. Colloidal silver is an excellent therapy for pink eye because the silver particles in it assist in destroying germs and reducing inflammation. A bacterial infection causes pink eye. However, it is essential to emphasize that colloidal silver should not be utilized in place of conventional medical treatment in any circumstance.

If you have pink eyes, you should get medical attention as soon as possible so that any potentially significant underlying problems may be ruled out. In addition to conventional medical therapy, using colloidal silver may assist in hastening the body's natural recovery process and lower the probability of developing issues.

Oral Hygiene

One of the many applications of the popular natural medicine known as colloidal silver is in the field of oral hygiene. Colloidal silver is a kind of silver that consists of very minute particles of silver that are suspended in a liquid. These silver particles possess antibacterial capabilities, which allow them to be effective against a wide variety of microorganisms, including viruses, bacteria, and fungi.

Colloidal silver, when used as a mouthwash, can help eliminate the harmful bacteria that contribute to the development of plaque and gingivitis. In addition, the anti-inflammatory properties of colloidal silver can assist in reducing inflammation and accelerating the healing process in the tissues of the mouth. As a consequence of this, it is a fantastic natural choice for maintaining the health and cleanliness of your mouth.

Ulcers caused by diabetes

For hundreds of years, colloidal silver has been utilized as a treatment for diabetic ulcers. Colloidal silver's antibacterial characteristics make it useful for treating a broad variety of microbiological infections, including those caused by bacteria, fungi, and viruses. Because of this, it is an excellent therapy for infected wounds, particularly ulcers caused by diabetes.

Colloidal silver, in addition to its ability to eliminate dangerous infections, also has the potential to lessen inflammation and hasten the body's natural recovery process. Colloidal silver may be a viable choice for treating diabetic ulcers; however, further study is required to prove the efficiency of this treatment approach.

Gut cleansing

Recent years have seen a meteoric rise in the amount of interest in colloidal silver as a result of the potential benefits it possesses in the areas of gut health and cleansing. It is believed that colloidal silver possesses antibacterial properties, which makes it an ideal choice for eliminating dangerous bacteria that can lead to digestive disturbances. In addition, it has anti-inflammatory properties, which may help reduce inflammation in the intestines and speed up the healing process in the tissues.

Sanitizer

Colloidal silver may also be used as an antibacterial sanitizer, which is another possible application for this substance. It is purportedly effective against a broad variety of germs, including E. coli, salmonella, and staphylococcus, among others. Even MRSA, a kind of bacteria that is resistant to antibiotics, may be killed by colloidal silver, according to scientific research.

Skincare and wound care

Colloidal silver is most generally recognized for its use as an immunostimulant and antibacterial; however, there is some evidence that it may also have advantages for the treatment of skin conditions and wounds. Colloidal silver is purported to hasten the healing process and protect against infection when administered topically.

In addition to that, it is occasionally utilized as a natural remedy for acne and many other skin ailments. However, further study is required to validate the usefulness of colloidal silver in cosmetic applications involving the skin. Colloidal silver does not pose a significant health risk when used correctly; nonetheless, some individuals may experience skin irritation from its usage. If you are thinking about utilizing colloidal silver for your skin, you should first consult with a qualified medical expert.

The health of the hair and scalp

Some people feel that colloidal silver can help treat dandruff, dry scalp, and other disorders that affect the scalp. In addition, some people use colloidal silver as a natural treatment for their hair to give it luster and make it feel softer. Some people feel that the use of colloidal silver can be good for the health of their hair and scalp, even though there is no scientific proof to back these claims. If you are interested in learning more about the benefits of using colloidal silver for your hair or scalp, you should consult with either your primary care physician or a professional cosmetologist.

Foot infections

Infections of the foot, such as athletes' feet and various forms of nail fungus, are common disorders that are sometimes challenging to eliminate. Colloidal silver, on the other hand, possesses antifungal qualities, which provide it an excellent therapy for the aforementioned illnesses. Nobody likes having stinky feet, but happily, stinky feet are another problem that colloidal silver may help with. Because it possesses antibacterial characteristics, it can eliminate the germs that are responsible for the foul odor that comes from sweaty feet.

Cancer treatment

Colloidal silver may potentially be useful in the treatment of cancer, according to the findings of some research. Colloidal silver has been demonstrated to be effective in killing cancer cells when used in vitro. Cancer is a disease that is defined by the abnormal development of cells (in a laboratory setting). However, to identify whether or not colloidal silver is a successful treatment for cancer in humans, further study is required.

Prevents food spoilage

Colloidal silver is another option for preventing food from going bad, as it contains antibacterial properties. It has been discovered to either slow down or inhibit the growth of germs on food products, which may aid in keeping such foods preserved for extended periods. This is because colloidal silver eradicates the bacteria that are responsible for the production of toxins and the contamination of food.

Cleaning agents

Colloidal silver may be used by homeowners to manufacture homemade cleaning products that are both safe and effective. Because it has antibacterial properties, it may be used to clean surfaces that are contaminated with germs, bacteria, and other potentially hazardous things.

In addition, because it is non-toxic, unlike many other cleaning solutions that are based on chemicals, it will not harm the environment or your health in any way. Colloidal silver is an excellent natural cleaning agent because of its ability to eliminate odors and prevent the growth of mold, mildew, and fungi. In addition, it can kill mold, mildew, and fungi.

It is essential to point out that although a great number of individuals are persuaded of the health advantages of colloidal silver, there is, as of yet, no proof that can definitively validate the claims that have been made about it. Before taking colloidal silver, you should always get the advice of a qualified medical practitioner, and you should never consume excessive amounts of it or use it for an extended length of time. Colloidal silver should also be avoided by people who are currently suffering from several pre-existing medical issues.

Potential Risks and Side Effects of Colloidal Silver

There is no evidence to support the claims that colloidal silver is an effective therapy for any ailment, even though it is advertised as a nutritional supplement and sold in stores. The use of colloidal silver over an extended period may result in major adverse health effects:

Argyria

Argyria is a disorder in which the skin appears blue or gray, and it is the most well-known adverse reaction to colloidal silver. Argyria is also the name of the condition. Argyria is a condition that develops when there is an accumulation of silver particles in the tissues of the body.

This is something that can occur if a person consumes significant quantities of colloidal silver over a prolonged period. In some people, argyria might last for the rest of their lives. Argyria is a condition that, in addition to discoloring the skin, can also cause an eclipse of the cornea, decreased sensitivity to light, and damage to the internal organs.

Headaches

Colloidal silver is a popular supplement that is often claimed for the therapeutic capabilities that it possesses. It is typically used to treat headaches. However, there is new evidence suggesting that it may cause headaches in some people. This might be because colloidal silver is a mineral, and just like any other mineral, it has the potential to induce an electrolyte imbalance.

Headaches and other symptoms are common outcomes of an electrolyte imbalance, which can also affect other bodily functions. If you use colloidal silver and find that it gives you headaches, you should stop taking it and talk to a doctor about the problem. You may evaluate whether or not your headaches are caused by colloidal silver with their assistance, and then choose a therapy that is both safer and more effective for you.

Injury to the Kidneys

Another possible side effect of using colloidal silver is kidney injury. It is the job of the kidneys to clean the blood and get rid of waste items that have accumulated throughout the body. When silver accumulates in the blood, it can cause damage to the kidneys and cause them to operate less efficiently. This can lead to several potentially serious health problems. Damage to the kidneys can, in extreme circumstances, result in renal failure, which can be deadly. Because of this, it is essential to be informed of the possible dangers of consuming colloidal silver and to speak with a healthcare professional before beginning any new supplement routine.

Injury to the Liver

The liver is a highly essential organ in the body, and it can sustain injury if colloidal silver is used for an extended period. When the liver is overburdened with silver particles, it is unable to function effectively and may sustain damage over time. The liver plays an important role in the elimination of harmful poisons from the body. A broad variety of symptoms, such as lethargy, nausea, vomiting, jaundice, and abdominal discomfort, can be brought on by injury to the liver.

Effects on the Nervous System

Colloidal silver can also influence the nervous system. Both epileptic seizures and neuropathy have been associated with exposure to colloidal silver. A disorder known as neuropathy damages nerves and can result in pain, numbness, and tingling in the limbs. Neuropathy can also be caused by diabetes. In extreme circumstances, it may result in paralysis.

An association between epileptic seizures and exposure to colloidal silver has also been found. Electrical abnormalities in the brain can occur suddenly and cannot be regulated, and this can lead to seizures. They have the potential to bring on convulsions, as well as spasms of the muscles and loss of consciousness. Both of these illnesses have the potential to be severe, and one of them may even be fatal.

Drug Interactions

A possible risk associated with colloidal silver is the possibility of adverse drug interactions. Colloidal silver's potential to interact negatively with other treatments, such as antibiotics, has the potential to lessen the effectiveness of those other medications. Before taking any drug, whether it be colloidal silver or something else, it is essential to be informed of the possible risks involved and to discuss the matter with a trained medical practitioner.

Nausea, vomiting, and diarrhea

Colloidal silver is a well-liked alternative treatment that has gained popularity due to claims that it may alleviate a variety of unpleasant symptoms, including nausea, vomiting, and diarrhea. On the other hand, it can induce several adverse effects, such as nausea, vomiting, and diarrhea. When used in high amounts or over an extended period, colloidal silver is associated with a higher risk of causing negative effects like these. If you use colloidal silver and have any of these adverse effects, you should speak with your healthcare physician as soon as possible. They may be able to suggest an alternative treatment choice that will work better for someone like you.

Silver allergy

If you believe that you may have a silver allergy, you must consult with a medical professional before using colloidal silver. Redness, swelling, itching, and hives are some of the symptoms that might accompany a silver allergy. In really severe instances, an allergy to silver might potentially cause respiratory difficulties. Even if you do have an allergy to silver, there are a great many different treatment choices available to you for the problem. Your physician will be able to guide you in the direction of the treatment that is most appropriate for your unique circumstances.

May cause the bone to release calcium

The use of colloidal silver for an extended period may cause bones to release calcium, which can lead to bones that are more brittle and fragile. Calcium is essential to the health, strength, and pliability of bones, and appropriate levels of calcium are required. To preserve good bone health, an individual needs to keep the calcium levels in their body at the appropriate amounts. If you want to use colloidal silver for a lengthy period, it is vital to have your bone density checked regularly and to take a calcium supplement if one is recommended for you.

It is essential to point out that antibiotics and other tried-and-true medical therapies should not be substituted with colloidal silver as a therapy for illness. An excess of colloidal silver can cause severe adverse effects on one's health.

Before beginning treatment with colloidal silver, it is essential to have a conversation with your primary care provider. It is possible that, in certain circumstances, it might be an advantageous adjunct to conventional medical therapy for certain disorders. However, as a treatment for any ailment or condition by itself, it is not advised as a stand-alone therapy in most cases.

Who should not use colloidal silver?

The use of colloidal silver as a complementary or alternative treatment has a long and illustrious history. However, anyone who has a history of renal illness, pregnant women, children younger than six years old, and anybody who is allergic to silver should not use colloidal silver. Other persons who should avoid using colloidal silver include those who are allergic to silver. A deeper look will now be taken at each of these categories of persons.

People who have a history of renal disease

Those who have a history of kidney disease should steer clear of using colloidal silver since it has the potential to cause more harm to the kidneys. Colloidal silver, in particular, has the potential to build up in the kidneys, which can ultimately result in renal failure.

In addition, colloidal silver has the potential to interact negatively with some drugs that are prescribed for the treatment of renal disease, rendering such medications less effective. Because of this, those who have renal issues should steer clear of utilizing colloidal silver and instead see their physician about other ways to enhance their health.

Pregnant women

Colloidal silver should not be used by pregnant women since it has the potential to cause several harmful side effects, and pregnant women should avoid using it. Silver is a metal, and as such, it can pass through the placenta and accumulate in the developing embryo. This is important to keep in mind. This might result in a disease known as argyria, which gives the skin a bluish-gray coloration and can be quite unpleasant.

In addition to this, silver has been shown to inhibit the body's ability to absorb critical nutrients, which can lead to developmental issues in the unborn child. Because the FDA does not regulate colloidal silver, there is no way to determine whether or not it is safe to use while pregnant. This brings us to our final point. Because of these concerns, it is not recommended that pregnant women use colloidal silver.

Children under the age of six

Colloidal silver may also produce major adverse consequences, particularly in children less than six years old. This is especially true in the case of children who are younger than six years old. Youngsters in this age range are more sensitive to the negative effects of colloidal silver than other children since their bodies are still developing at this point.

Problems with the digestive system, anemia, and harm to the central nervous system are all possible outcomes of these adverse effects. Because of these risks, it is essential to discuss the use of colloidal silver with a medical professional before administering it to a kid who is less than six years old.

People who are allergic to silver

People who are allergic to silver should be informed that colloidal silver can trigger an allergic reaction in those with silver sensitivity. It is crucial to be aware of this possibility. The most typical manifestation of sensitivity to silver is contact dermatitis, a skin condition that is characterized by redness, itchiness, and inflammation.

Colloidal silver has the potential to produce anaphylaxis, a severe allergic reaction that might be fatal in extreme situations. If you have an allergy to silver, the most crucial thing for you to do is to stay away from products that contain silver in any form, including colloidal silver. If you have used a product that contains silver and are experiencing any symptoms, you should get medical assistance as soon as possible.

In conclusion, even though colloidal silver is a kind of complementary and alternative medicine that has been utilized for millennia, some individuals can have major adverse effects from using it. It is strongly recommended that you do not use colloidal silver if you are in any of the aforementioned groups.

However, if you are otherwise healthy and do not suffer from any allergies, you might want to give colloidal silver a go as an alternate kind of treatment. Just be sure to see your physician first, and then make sure to strictly adhere to their dosage instructions.

Government's Reactions to Colloidal Silver

In August of 1999, the Food and Drug Administration (FDA) of the United States of America issued a judgment that made it illegal for sellers of colloidal silver to make any claims regarding the product's efficacy as a medicine. This ruling prevented sellers from making any claims about the product's ability to treat or prevent disease. If a pharmaceutical has not been subjected to the stringent testing for both safety and efficacy that is required of medications, then it is impossible to claim that taking that medication has any positive medical effects.

Because colloidal silver has not been put through these sorts of studies, the Food and Drug Administration in the United States accepts it as a dietary supplement (dietary supplements cannot claim to cure diseases, only that they "support healthy functioning"). The Food and Drug Administration has issued warnings to websites that are selling or marketing colloidal silver as an antibiotic or for other therapeutic applications online.

These websites may be found by searching "Food and Drug Administration warning websites." If there are no supposed health benefits linked with the use of colloidal silver, it is advertised as a dietary supplement. The distribution of colloidal silver is not against the law so long as the product in issue is by all of the FDA's other regulations.

In 2002, the Australian Therapeutic Goods Administration issued a ruling in which it stated that products containing colloidal silver were no longer exempt from the therapeutic goods legislation and that these products were required to meet the requirements of other products that were covered by this law. The ruling also stated that the exemption for these products from the legislation had been removed. The decision to issue the judgment was made because the administration thought that the standards for these items were not being satisfied adequately.

An investigation conducted by the TGA concluded that "there are no current legitimate uses of colloidal silver." As a result of this finding, the TGA recommended that the Surveillance Section of the TGA be asked to investigate the illegal availability of colloidal silver products due to concerns regarding the high toxicity of these products. The following is a list of some of the reasons why it was advised that you do this:

"There is little evidence to support therapeutic claims made for colloidal silver products; the risk to consumers of silver toxicity outweighs the value of trying an unsubstantiated treatment, and bacterial resistance to silver can occur." [T]here is little evidence to support therapeutic claims made for colloidal silver products. Because it poses a substantial risk to public health, the availability of items containing illegally produced colloidal silver should be restricted via concerted efforts.

Conclusion

Colloidal silver is a natural medicine that has been used for a variety of illnesses for ages. It is effective. Even while there is some indication that it may have potential advantages, there are still a lot of studies that need to be done before we can have a complete understanding of the product's safety and how well it works.

Conventional and more up-to-date variants of colloidal silver are both now on the market; nevertheless, the precise mechanism of action of each type of colloidal silver is still a mystery. Although it can have potential hazards and side effects, these are likely to vary based not just on how a person reacts to the product, but also on the concentration of the product and how it is administered.

Before using colloidal silver, those with certain medical issues or those who are currently on medication should always consult with their primary care physician. Even though there have been some debates over its usage, it is still widely used today even though several governments throughout the world have made measures to restrict its access and use.

Those individuals who are interested in investigating natural options for coping with health difficulties may perhaps find this interesting. To answer this question, however, further research into the efficacy and safety of colloidal silver is required. Only then will it be possible to identify whether or not it can be of use in the treatment of common disorders.

In the end, if you want to enhance your general health and wellness without resorting to ingesting colloidal silver, you may do it naturally in several other ways as well. Consuming nutritious foods, engaging in physically active pursuits regularly, and obtaining sufficient amounts of sleep are all essential components of establishing and sustaining a healthy lifestyle.

Before beginning the use of any new goods or therapies, it is advisable to speak with a trained medical practitioner if you have any reason to believe that colloidal silver might be useful to your health. They will be able to offer guidance and information on the potential dangers and advantages linked with the usage of colloidal silver. They will also be able to advise on the potential risks.

In addition, they will be able to provide suggestions for any other modifications to your way of life that may better support your overall health. In the end, we can all live vibrant lives that are full of energy and well-being if we make responsible decisions that are based on the advice of experts and engage in healthy activities such as eating meals that are rich in nutrients and exercising regularly.

FAQ About Colloidal Silver

1. What is colloidal silver?

A solution of silver particles in water is what we refer to as colloidal silver. Since ancient times, it has been employed as an antibacterial agent, and in more recent times, it has gained popularity as an alternative therapy for a wide range of illnesses.

2. How does it work?

Colloidal silver is effective because it inhibits the reproduction of bacteria, viruses, and fungi by binding to the proteins found in these pathogens. Because of this property, it is an efficient antibacterial agent.

3. What are the benefits of colloidal silver?

The power of colloidal silver to destroy bacteria, viruses, and fungi, as well as its anti-inflammatory characteristics and ability to enhance the immune system, are three of the many advantages of using this substance. In addition, the use of colloidal silver as a treatment for illnesses such as acne, sinus infections, and ear infections has shown promising results.

4. Are there any side effects?

The disorder known as argyria, which causes the skin to develop a bluish-gray color, is the adverse reaction to colloidal silver that occurs the most frequently. Argyria is uncommon and almost often results from the consistent use of large amounts of colloidal silver over an extended period. In addition to stomach distress, headaches, and dizziness may also occur as possible side effects.

5. How do I take colloidal silver?

Oral consumption or topical use of colloidal silver are also viable options. When ingesting colloidal silver through the oral route, it is essential to begin treatment with a modest dose and progressively increase it as directed. When using colloidal silver for a topical application, you have the option of putting it straight to the skin or incorporating it into a lotion or cream.

6. Where can I buy colloidal silver?

Colloidal silver is available for purchase in various health food stores and even on the internet. It is essential to make certain that you acquire your colloidal silver from a trustworthy supplier if you want to be certain that the product you buy is of a superior grade.

References and Helpful Links

"A Silver Bullet against MRSA: Silver Ion-Coated Medical Devices Could Fight MRSA While Creating New Bone." ScienceDaily, https://www.sciencedaily.com/releases/2017/02/170208193632.htm. Accessed 13 Feb. 2023.

"Colloidal Silver." NCCIH, https://www.nccih.nih.gov/health/colloidal-silver. Accessed 13 Feb. 2023.

Colloidal Silver For Preserving And Healing – Ziemia. https://ziemia.life/colloidal-silver/. Accessed 13 Feb. 2023.

"Colloidal Silver: Uses, Safety, and Side Effects." Healthline, 19 Jan. 2022, https://www.healthline.com/nutrition/colloidal-silver.

"History of Silver." Sovereign Silver, https://sovereignsilver.com/pages/history-of-silver. Accessed 13 Feb. 2023.

"Is Colloidal Silver Safe and Effective?" Cleveland Clinic, 3 Mar. 2022, https://health.clevelandclinic.org/is-colloidal-silver-safe/.

"What Is Colloidal Silver?" Verywell Health, https://www.verywellhealth.com/colloidal-silver-what-you-need-to-know-89555. Accessed 13 Feb. 2023.

www.ingramcontent.com/pod-product-compliance
Lightning Source LLC
LaVergne TN
LVHW010437070526
838199LV00066B/6056